Praise for

Every Woman's Battle and *Every Young Woman's Battle*
by Shannon Ethridge

"There is a common, almost Victorian, myth that women don't really struggle with sexual sin. That myth causes many women to feel a double shame. The shame of struggling sexually is compounded by the assumption that few, if any, women share the same battle. Shannon Ethridge artfully and boldly unveils the war and offers women a way to enter the battle with courage, hope, and grace. *Every Woman's Battle* will help both men and women comprehend the glorious beauty and sensuality of holiness. This is a desperately needed book."

—DAN B. ALLENDER, PhD, president of Mars Hill Graduate
School and author of *The Healing Path*

"This book sheds light on the often unspoken sensitivities and issues that women wrestle with. Not only is it well written, it is liberating and refreshing, with sound principles for overcoming the things that threaten to keep us from experiencing the fullness of joy that is part of God's big picture plan for our lives."

—MICHELLE MCKINNEY HAMMOND, author of *Get Over It
and On With It*

"A 'powerful shield' for every woman. Shannon's words are convicting, challenging, and confronting."

—DR. TIM CLINTON, president of the American Association
of Christian Counselors

"Many of my *Bad Girls of the Bible* readers have tearfully confessed to me their struggles with sexual sins—promiscuity, adultery, and self-gratification among them. Since we cannot pretend Christian women don't face these temptations, it's a relief to have a sound resource like this one to recommend. Shannon Ethridge's straightforward, nonjudgmental, step-by-step approach can help women 'come clean' in the best way possible—through an intimate relationship with the Lover of their souls."

—LIZ CURTIS HIGGS, best-selling author of *Bad Girls of the Bible,*
Really Bad Girls of the Bible, and *Mad Mary: A Bad Girl from*
Magdala

"If you're like me, you are going to find Shannon's book immeasurably helpful. *Every Woman's Battle* is the best resource I know for embracing God's plan of sexual and emotional integrity as a woman."

—LESLIE PARROTT, author of *When Bad Things Happen*
to Good Marriages

every single woman's battle

Shannon Ethridge

every single woman's battle

Guarding Your Heart and Mind Against Sexual and Emotional Compromise

A Companion Guide for Personal or Group Study

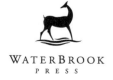

WATERBROOK
PRESS

EVERY SINGLE WOMAN'S BATTLE
PUBLISHED BY WATERBROOK PRESS
2375 Telstar Drive, Suite 160
Colorado Springs, Colorado 80920
A division of Random House Inc.

Quotations from *Every Woman's Battle* © 2003 by Shannon Ethridge and *Every Man's Battle* © 2000 by Stephen Arterburn, Fred Stoeker, and Mike Yorkey.

All Scripture quotations, unless otherwise indicated, are taken from the *Holy Bible, New International Version*®. NIV®. Copyright © 1973, 1978, 1984 by International Bible Society. Used by permission of Zondervan Publishing House. All rights reserved. Scripture quotations marked (KJV) are taken from the *King James Version*. Scripture quotations marked (MSG) are taken from *The Message*. Copyright © 1993, 1994, 1995, 1996, 2000, 2001, 2002. Used by permission of NavPress Publishing Group. Scripture quotations marked (RSV) are taken from the *Revised Standard Version of the Bible,* copyright © 1946, 1952, and 1971 by the Division of Christian Education of the National Council of the Churches of Christ in the USA. Used by permission.

Names and facts from stories contained in this book have been changed, but the emotional and sexual struggles portrayed are true stories as related to the author through personal interviews, letters, or e-mails.

ISBN 1-4000-7127-5

Published in association with the literary agency of Alive Communications Inc., 7680 Goddard Street, Suite 200, Colorado Springs, CO 80920.

Printed in the United States of America
2005—First Edition

10 9 8 7 6 5 4 3 2 1

contents

questions you may have about this workbook

What will *Every Single Woman's Battle* do for me?

Living a life of sexual integrity as a single woman is so much more than refraining from intercourse. And it certainly is not about removing pleasure from your life. This workbook will address the real temptations you face, help you evaluate the lifestyle you have chosen thus far, and teach you to build into your daily life natural and enjoyable ways of fulfilling your God-given desires.

Is this workbook enough or do I also need the book *Every Woman's Battle*?

Included in the studies you'll find excerpts from *Every Woman's Battle* (marked at beginning and end with this symbol: 📚) and from *Every Man's Battle* (marked at beginning and end by this symbol: 📖). These excerpts were chosen because of how they apply specifically to the life of a single woman, but they also offer wisdom for issues that women in general face. Although it would be beneficial for you to read *Every Woman's Battle,* you will find this book adequate to help you journey toward sexual integrity.

How much time is required? Do I need to work through every part of each chapter?

Seeking sexual and emotional fulfillment is an important endeavor. If your purpose in using the book is group discussion, you can expect to spend an hour each week to prepare for the group meeting; however, some people spend as little as a half hour, and others spend several hours. The amount of time you invest depends on how deeply you want to probe into your heart on this issue.

Prior to meeting with the group, you should take time to read the chapter, highlighting important concepts and jotting down personal responses or ideas; answer the personal questions, praying often for insight and grace; read the questions the group will discuss, searching your heart so that you will not be caught unaware if a certain topic opens old wounds.

This workbook is designed to promote your thorough exploration of the content, but you may find it best to focus your time and discussion on some sections and questions more than others.

How do I find a study group?

If your church or Christian organization does not already have a small-group meeting to discuss this topic, start one yourself. As facilitator, you simply need to have an authentic and nonjudgmental attitude. The questions offered in the workbook are clear, and no one will expect you to have all the answers. If you regularly encourage the women to participate in the discussion with honesty and desire for growth, you will find that everyone will have something of value to add. Note that you will occasionally have to redirect the conversation to make sure that everyone stays on track and that each woman is given an opportunity to contribute to the conversation.

The workbook is set up so you complete one lesson per week and finish in eight weeks. The study can also be expanded to twelve weeks if you prefer—you would choose four of the lessons and study each one over a two-week period instead of each one over a single week. (You would study the remaining four lessons over a one-week period each.) Another option would be to read a single chapter a week (for twelve weeks) from *Every Woman's Battle,* following along accordingly in this workbook.

Each of your meetings could happen during a lunch hour at work, in the early morning before work begins, on a weekday evening, or even a Sunday morning. Open the meetings up to any single woman who treasures the idea of being part of a deep spiritual community and who can promise to give and receive grace and truth.

The study can also be used in a mixed-gender small group. This type of combined discussion can help both women and men see the similarities in their journeys, as well as gain greater understanding of their differences.

If you have been wandering in the disappointing world of what was and what might have been, *Every Woman's Battle* will bring you back to the reality of what God wants you to be.... I pray that when you are finished reading you will be on a path of spiritual growth and maturity that will allow you to stand pure before the Lord....

May God bless you greatly for your desire to seek His truth.

—from the foreword to *Every Woman's Battle*

Take heart and know that your cries for help have been heard. This book is a training manual that will help you avoid sexual and emotional compromise and will show you how to experience God's plan for sexual and emotional fulfillment.... Do you want to be a woman of sexual and emotional integrity? With God's help you can. Let's get started.

—from the introduction to *Every Woman's Battle*

whose battle is it?

At one time I was having extramarital affairs with five different men.... Even though I wasn't having sexual intercourse with any of these other men, I was still having an affair with each of them—a mental and/or emotional affair. My fantasies of being Clark Gable's leading lady, memories of my romantic relationship with Ray, and fascination with Tom's wit, Mark's maturity, and Scott's verbal talents affected my marriage in a way just as damaging as a sexual affair would have.

When I hear people say that women don't struggle with sexual issues like men do, I cannot help but wonder what planet they are from or what rock they have been hiding under. Perhaps what they really mean is, the *physical* act of sex isn't an overwhelming temptation for women like it is for men.

Men and women struggle in different ways when it comes to sexual integrity. While a man's battle begins with what he takes in through his eyes, a woman's begins with her heart and her thoughts. A man must guard his eyes to maintain sexual integrity, but because God made women to be emotionally and mentally stimulated, we must closely guard our hearts and minds as well as our bodies if we want to experience God's plan for sexual and emotional fulfillment. A woman's battle is for sexual *and* emotional integrity. ☕

☕ Paul understood our very human tendency to live in denial, closing our eyes to the things in our lives that may need to change. Change is hard work, and we would rather stay as we are. But this is not how God has called us to live. He wants to help us control our minds and our desires so that we can be more like Him. He wants to help us discover His plan for relational satisfaction. But we can't do this if we insist on keeping our eyes closed to the compromise that robs us of ultimate sexual and emotional fulfillment. ☕

PLANTING GOOD SEEDS
(Personally Seeking God's Truth)

1. How important is the Word of God to you? Why?

As you seek to discover God's plan for sexual and emotional fulfillment, plant these good seeds in your heart:

The one who sows to please his sinful nature, from that nature will reap destruction; the one who sows to please the Spirit, from the Spirit will reap eternal life. (Galatians 6:8)

Each one is tempted when, by his own evil desire, he is dragged away and enticed. Then, after desire has conceived, it gives birth to sin; and sin, when it is full-grown, gives birth to death. (James 1:14-15)

2.   What, if anything, in these verses feels like a threat or a warning to you? Why do you think you respond to the verses the way you do?

To increase your hope of winning the battle for sexual and emotional integrity, plant this good seed from 1 Corinthians 10:13 in your heart:

No temptation has seized you except what is common to [woman]. And God is faithful; he will not let you be tempted beyond what you can bear. But when you are tempted, he will also provide a way out so that you can stand up under it.

3.   What does this promise mean to you?

WEEDING OUT DECEPTION
(Recognizing the Truth)

In some way or another sexual and emotional integrity is a battle that every woman fights. However, many women are fighting this battle with their eyes closed because they don't believe they are even engaged in the battle. Many believe that just because they are not involved in a physical, sexual affair, they don't have a problem with sexual and emotional integrity. As a result, they engage in thoughts and behaviors that compromise their integrity and rob them of true sexual and emotional fulfillment.

4. Do you agree with the statement that every woman fights the battle for sexual and emotional integrity? On what do you base your opinion?

5. The author warns that it is not wise to think that sexual immorality can't happen to any one of us. How prevalent do you think sexual immorality is among Christian singles?

6. Circle how often you have engaged in any of the following:

Unhealthy Comparisons	Never	Sometimes	Often	Always
Mental Fantasies	Never	Sometimes	Often	Always
Emotional Affairs	Never	Sometimes	Often	Always
Romance Novels	Never	Sometimes	Often	Always
Soap Operas	Never	Sometimes	Often	Always
Masturbation	Never	Sometimes	Often	Always
Inappropriate Internet Activity	Never	Sometimes	Often	Always
Other Sexual Dysfunction(s)	Never	Sometimes	Often	Always

To determine if you are engaged in the battle for sexual and emotional integrity, answer the following questions adapted from *Every Woman's Battle*.

	Yes/No
Is having a man in your life or finding a husband something that dominates your thoughts?	_____
If you have a man in your life, do you compare him to other men (physically, mentally, emotionally, or spiritually)?	_____
Do you often obsess over who the "next man" in your life could be?	_____
Do you have sexual secrets that you don't want anyone else to know about?	_____

Do you feel like a nobody if you don't have a love interest
in your life? Does a romantic relationship give you a sense
of identity?   _____

Do you seem to attract bad or dysfunctional relationships
with men?   _____

Do men accuse you of being manipulative or controlling?   _____

Do you feel secretly excited or powerful when you sense that
a man finds you attractive?   _____

Is remaining emotionally or physically faithful to one person
a challenge for you?   _____

Do you often choose your attire in the morning based on
the men you will encounter that day?   _____

Do you find yourself flirting or using sexual innuendos
(even if you do not intend to) when conversing with
someone you find attractive?   _____

Do you have to masturbate when you get sexually
aroused?   _____

Do you read romance novels because of the fantasies
they evoke within you or because they arouse you
sexually?   _____

Have you ever used premarital or extramarital relationships
to "medicate" your emotional pain?   _____

Is there any area of your sexuality that you would not want
your future husband to know about?   _____

Do you use pornography—either alone or with a
partner?   _____

Do you have a problem making and maintaining close
female friends?   _____

Do you converse with strangers in Internet chat rooms?   _____

Have you ever been unable to concentrate on work, school,
    or the affairs of your household because of thoughts or feel-
    ings you are having about someone else?   _____
Do you think the word *victim* describes you?   _____

7. What surprised you about your own answers? What scared
    you?

8. What particular question(s) hit home for you, and why?

9. Specifically, what effects have these types of activities had on your
    relationships with men? on your relationship with God? on your
    self-esteem?

☕ By definition, our sexuality isn't *what we do.* Even people who are committed to celibacy are sexual beings. Our sexuality is *who we are,* and we were made with a body, mind, heart, and spirit, not just a body. Therefore, sexual integrity is not just about physical chastity. It is about purity in all four aspects of our being (body, mind, heart, and spirit). When all four aspects line up perfectly, our "tabletop" (our life) reflects balance and integrity.… [See illustration on next page.] ☕

☕ It's no laughing matter when one of the "legs" of our sexuality buckles, because then our lives can become slippery slopes leading to discontentment, sexual compromise, self-loathing, and emotional brokenness. When this happens, the blessing that God intended to bring richness and pleasure to our lives feels more like a curse that brings great pain and despair. ☕

10. In your dating relationships, where have you set "the line" of sexual integrity? How far is it "okay" to go prior to marriage? Where does this belief come from?

11. If you ever crossed that imaginary line, were you able to back up and reestablish your previous standards? How did you do it or fail to do it?

🎺 HARVESTING FULFILLMENT
(Applying the Truth)

📖 God...wants to help us control our minds and our desires so that we can be more like Him. He wants to help us discover His plan for relational satisfaction. But we can't do this if we insist on keeping our eyes closed to the compromise that robs us of ultimate sexual and emotional fulfillment. 📖

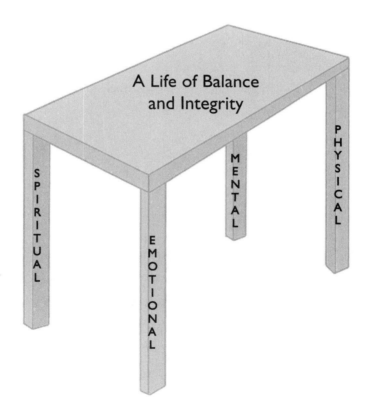

12. If you were to allow God to control your mind and desires, what would be the result in regard to your love life? your relationship with God? your self-esteem?

🌿 GROWING TOGETHER
(Sharing the Truth in Small-Group Discussion)

13. What prompted you to pick up *Every Single Woman's Battle?* What is the main thing you are hoping to gain over the next eight weeks as you read this book? as you participate in this discussion group?

🍵 While a man needs mental, emotional, and spiritual connection, his physical needs tend to be in the driver's seat and his other needs ride along in the back. The reverse is true for women. If there is one particular need that drives us, it is certainly our emotional needs. That's why it's said that men *give love to get sex* and women *give sex to get love.* 🍵

14. Have you ever engaged in any form of sexual activity in order to get the love you were longing for? If so, did you get the desired result? How did the result affirm or challenge your behavior?

15. Obviously women have sexual needs as well as emotional needs. Have you ever felt you should not experience sexual desires? If so, how did that make you feel? Why?

16. What other beliefs about sexuality have shaped your emotions and behaviors around this topic? How do you discern which beliefs are false and which are true?

17. Do you think it is more difficult for men than for women to maintain sexual integrity? Why or why not?

18. Do you think it is more difficult for single women than for married women to maintain sexual integrity? Why or why not?

19. Does discussing the sexual temptations you face with mature, caring adults help you maintain sexual integrity? Why or why not? If not, what would help?

For a Christian woman, sexual and emotional integrity means that her thoughts, words, emotions, and actions all reflect an inner beauty and a sincere love for God, others, and herself. This doesn't mean she is never tempted to think, say, feel, or do something inappropriate, but that she tries diligently to resist these temptations and stands firm in her convictions. She doesn't use men in an attempt to get her emotional cravings met or entertain sexual or romantic fantasies about men she is not married to.... She doesn't dress to seek male attention, but she doesn't limit herself to a wardrobe of ankle-length muumuus, either. She may dress fashionably and look sharp or may even appear sexy (like beauty, sexy is in the eye of the beholder), but her motivation isn't self-seeking or seductive. She presents herself as an attractive woman because she knows she represents God to others.

20. When is striving to look beautiful a sin and when is it not? How can we best evaluate our own motivations?

21. Share your conclusions about what you see as your strengths and weaknesses when it comes to being a woman of sexual and emotional integrity.

Jehovah Jireh, I trust You for my every need. Please give me wisdom and courage as I seek emotional and sexual integrity. And above all, keep me connected to You—draw me ever closer—so that I may know where my true fulfillment comes from. Amen.

finding truth

 In my thirteen years of speaking and lay counseling with women on sexual issues, I've uncovered [five] popular myths that I believe confuse the issue and make sexual integrity far more challenging. Although at first glance you may not believe that you subscribe to a particular misconception, I encourage you to read about it anyway. We are often only aware of what we believe in regard to the things we have actually experienced but are undecided about our beliefs regarding the things or feelings we have not yet experienced. If we understand these myths and the lies they are based on, we'll have a stronger defense if and when we're tempted in one of these areas.

- There's nothing wrong with comparing myself or my [relationship] to other people.
- I am mature enough to watch any movie or television show, read any book, listen to any music, or surf any Web sites without being affected in a negative way.
- Masturbation does not hurt me, my relationship with my future husband, or my relationship with God.
- Because I feel so sexually tempted, I must already be guilty, so why bother resisting?
- There's no one who would really understand my struggle.

📖 When challenged by His higher standards, we're comforted that we don't look too different from those around us. Trouble is, we don't look much different from non-Christians either.

Our adolescent Christians are often indistinguishable from their non-Christian peers, sharing the same activities, music, jokes, and attitudes about premarital sex. Kristin, a teenager, told us, "Our youth group is filled with kids faking their Christian walk. They are actually taking drugs, drinking, partying, and having sex. If you want to walk purely, it's easier to hang around with the non-Christians at school than to hang around with the Christians at church. I say that because school friends know where I stand and they say, 'That's cool—I can accept that.' The Christian kids mock me, laughing and asking, 'Why be so straight? Get a life!' They pressure my values at every turn." She told us about Brad, a lay leader's son, who told her, "I know intercourse is wrong before marriage, but anything short of that is fine. I love to get up under a bra."

Sadly, the adults are no different from the Christian teens. Linda, a single career woman, says her adult singles group at church has "players"—men and women who stalk their prey to satisfy their own needs.... Have we gone blind? What can we expect from our across-the-board commitment to the middle ground? Don't we realize that our recent converts to Christianity will become just like us? Will it be a comfort to see them just as lazy regarding their personal devotion to Jesus as we are? 📖

📚 [The] pursuit of "love" takes the form of searching for intimacy and closeness, and unfortunately the world we live in teaches that this intimacy and closeness can be found only through sexual relationships. However, as many women have painfully discovered, relationships can be built entirely on sex and still be devoid of any intimacy or closeness at all, which leaves us feeling even more powerless to have our needs met.

Unfortunately, women have long been using sex in order to get their own needs met. In fact, this has been going on since biblical times. Paul preached against it in his first letter to Timothy when he wrote, "I do not permit a woman to teach or to have authority over a man; she must be silent" (2:12). Some people have interpreted this verse as an injunction to keep women from any form of leadership in the church, but I believe it has nothing to do with teaching the gospel or justly exercising her authority to lead others to Christ. As I've researched the actual Greek word that Paul was using for "authority," I have come to believe he was addressing the exact issue we're talking about in this chapter: *women using sex to exert power over men.*[1]

PLANTING GOOD SEEDS
(Personally Seeking God's Truth)

As you seek to discern the difference between myth and truth in your battle for sexual and emotional integrity, plant these good seeds in your heart:

> To the Jews who had believed him, Jesus said, "If you hold to my teaching, you are really my disciples. Then you will know the truth, and the truth will set you free." (John 8:31-32)

1. Has studying God's Word revealed truth to you, setting you free? What is that truth? From what were you set free?

---

1. Kari Torjesen Malcom, *Women at the Crossroads* (Downers Grove, Ill.: InterVarsity, 1982), 78–9.

> The good [woman] brings good things out of the good stored up in [her] heart, and the evil [woman] brings evil things out of the evil stored up in [her] heart. For out of the overflow of [her] heart [her] mouth speaks. (Luke 6:45)

2. What are you storing up in your heart? Describe how your thinking has spilled over into your words and actions.

As you realize your need for God's grace in these matters, plant this seed in your heart:

> For we do not have a high priest who is unable to sympathize with our weaknesses, but we have one who has been tempted in every way, just as we are—yet was without sin. Let us then approach the throne of grace with confidence, so that we may receive mercy and find grace to help us in our time of need. (Hebrews 4:15-16)

3. How does it make you feel to know that Jesus can sympathize with your every weakness (even your sexual weaknesses)? Explain your answer.

⚒ WEEDING OUT DECEPTION
(Recognizing the Truth)

☕ When we compare ourselves to others, we put one person above the other. We either come out on top (producing vanity and pride in our lives), or we come up short (producing feelings of disappointment with what God gave us). Regardless of how we measure up when we make these comparisons, our motives are selfish and sinful rather than loving. ☕

4. Do you spend time comparing yourself with other women? In what ways? What has been the result?

5. Do you often compare one man with another, expecting to find the perfect one? What has been the result?

☕ When we think about doing something and play it out in our thoughts, it makes it that much easier to engage in the behavior. If a woman cannot control herself while alone, what hope does she have when some smooth-talking hunk of a man starts whispering sweet nothings in her ear?

Also, no lust can ever be satisfied; once you begin feeding baby monsters, their appetites grow bigger and they require *more!* You are better off never feeding those monsters in the first place.

6. Do you ever fantasize about an activity that you believe is wrong? How can you protect yourself from acting out your thoughts?

7. If you masturbate, do you find yourself fulfilled by the activity or even more hungry for physical affection? Why do you think that is?

It is normal to feel attracted to multiple people. It is not normal to *attach* yourself to multiple people. Remember that love is not a feeling, but a commitment.

8. Do you usually act on your feelings of attraction? How can you discern between love and attraction?

📖 God holds *you* responsible, and if you don't gain control before your wedding day, you can expect it to crop up after the honeymoon. If you're single and watching sensual R-rated movies, wedded bliss won't change this habit. If your eyes lock on passing babes, they'll still roam after you say "I do." You're masturbating now? Putting that ring on your finger won't keep your hands off yourself. 📖

9. Do you expect marriage to eliminate all your sexual temptations? Why or why not? What sexual-temptation problems might be most difficult to overcome?

🐟 HARVESTING FULFILLMENT
(Applying the Truth)

📚 If we crave genuine intimacy, we must learn to seek it only in this kind of [a] grace-filled relationship. The word *intimacy* itself can be best defined by breaking it into syllables, *in-to-me-see.* Can we see into each other and respect, appreciate, and value what is really there, regardless of how that measures up to anyone else? That is what unconditional love and relational intimacy is all about, and this type of intimacy can be discovered only by two people who are seeking sexual and emotional integrity with all their mind, body, heart, and soul. 📚

10. Do you have any reservations about those closest to you seeing into every part of you? Why or why not? What, if anything, do you hide from those closest to you, and why?

11. How can you offer the same grace to others that God gives to you? What things might you need to accept in order to love someone unconditionally and unreservedly?

Getting to know God more intimately means, in part, learning how He feels about you and understanding the provisions He has made in order to satisfy your innermost desires to feel loved, needed, and powerful (a righteous form of power, not a manipulative one). This is a great way to discover who you really are—not as the world tries to program you to be, but as your Maker designed you to be. Once you allow God to correct your beliefs about yourself, those beliefs will begin driving your decisions, your behaviors will follow directly behind, and you will have victory in this battle against sexual compromise.

12. Perhaps you've heard people talk about God as a husband. Does it seem possible to you to be satisfied with God as your sole partner? Why or why not?

13. What does it mean to be intimate with God? Do you believe God is capable of satisfying your innermost desires? How do you think He can do this?

❧ GROWING TOGETHER
(Sharing the Truth in Small-Group Discussion)

Sixty-seven percent of all women will experience at least one or more premarital or extramarital affair in her lifetime.[1] That is the number of women who *give in* to these temptations. I believe the percentage is much higher (I'm guessing in the 90 percent range) of those women who simply experience the temptation to engage in premarital or extramarital affairs.

---

1. Tim Clinton, from a class titled "Counselor Professional Identity, Function and Ethics Videotape Course," External Degree Program, Liberty University, Lynchburg, Va. Used with permission.

14. Do you find this statistic surprising with regard to our whole society? with regard to the Christian community? Why or why not?

15. In what ways does culture positively and negatively shape our sexual thoughts and behaviors?

16. In what ways does a religious upbringing positively and negatively shape our views of sex?

Another reason women aren't as open about their sexual struggles is because of the humiliation that comes with giving sex in order to get love. Most women don't brag about the number of sexual partners they've had. That's because for a woman the relationship is the prize; the sex was simply the price she had to pay to get the prize. If she paid the price, but still didn't get the prize, there is an incredible amount of humiliation that comes with that. What woman wants to announce to the world her humiliation? 📖☙

17. Do you find it difficult to confide in other women on this or other topics? How can this group become a safe place for you?

18. Have you ever "lost the prize" (a relationship) after "paying the price" (physical intimacy)? How did you deal with the lost relationship and/or rejection?

📖 Excellence isn't the same as obedience or perfection. The search for excellence leaves us overwhelmingly vulnerable to snare after snare since it allows room for mixture. The search for obedience or perfection does not.

Excellence is a *mixed* standard, while obedience is a *fixed* standard. We want to shoot for the fixed standard. 📖

19. In your own words, explain the difference between excellence and perfection. Knowing that we will never be perfect, why is it important to continue striving in that direction?

20. How do you discern between real and false shame? Do you have shame over past sins? What would it look like in your life to fully accept God's forgiveness?

21. Christians often say that sex is a beautiful gift from God. Do you believe that? How does this belief translate into behavior, especially for single women?

*H*oly Spirit, thank You for Your guidance and Your presence. Please open the Word to me so that I may clearly discern how to live in a way that pleases You and also fulfills me. Amen.

taking thoughts captive

You are getting into a four-door car by yourself. It's late at night and you are in a rough neighborhood. In order to feel safe, what is the first thing you are going to do when you get in the car? Right. Lock the doors.

How many doors will you lock? You may think this is a silly question, but think about it. If you only locked one or two or even three of the doors, would you be safe? Of course not. All four doors must be locked to keep out an unwelcome intruder.

The same is true with keeping out unwelcome sexual temptations. These temptations can invade our lives and eventually give birth to sin in four ways. The thoughts we choose to entertain in our minds can influence us. The words we speak or the conversations we engage in can lure us down unrighteous, dangerous paths. So can the failure to guard our hearts from getting involved in unhealthy relationships. And when we allow our bodies to be in the wrong place at the wrong time with the wrong person, we can be led toward sexual compromise.

Even if we leave only one of these doors unlocked, we are vulnerable. We must guard all four areas (our minds, our hearts, our mouths, and our bodies) to have any hope of remaining safe and maintaining sexual integrity.

📖 Our heavenly Father…wants us to be like Him. When He calls us to "be perfect as your Father in heaven is perfect," He's asking us to rise above our natural tendencies to impure eyes, fanciful minds, and wandering hearts. His standard of purity doesn't come naturally to us. He calls us to rise up, by the power of His indwelling presence, and get the job done.

Before an important battle for the army he commanded, Joab said to the troops of Israel, "Be of good courage, and let us play the men for our people" (2 Samuel 10:12, KJV). In short, he was saying, "We know God's plan for us. Let's rise up as men, and set our hearts and minds to get it done!"

Regarding sexual integrity, God wants *you* to rise up and get it done. 📖

🪣 PLANTING GOOD SEEDS
(Personally Seeking God's Truth)

Recognizing that the battle for sexual and emotional integrity begins in the mind, plant this good seed, 2 Corinthians 10:3-5, in your heart:

> For though we live in the world, we do not wage war as the world does. The weapons we fight with are not the weapons of the world…. We take captive every thought to make it obedient to Christ.

1. How is taking thoughts captive a weapon against sexual and emotional compromise? Is it a weapon you've learned to use effectively? If so, how? If not, how might you do so in the future?

As a guard against pursuing sexual and emotional fulfillment the world's way, plant the good seed of Romans 12:1-2 in your heart:

> Therefore, I urge you, [sisters], in view of God's mercy, to offer your bodies as living sacrifices, holy and pleasing to God—this is your spiritual act of worship. Do not conform any longer to the pattern of this world, but be transformed by the renewing of your mind. Then you will be able to test and approve what God's will is—his good, pleasing and perfect will.

2. Does God's generous mercy tend to draw you into righteous living? Or do you tend to use it as an excuse to pursue personal desires? Explain.

3. How will you "test and approve" what God's will is? (For help, consider Romans 12:2 from *The Message:* "Don't become so well-adjusted to your culture that you fit into it without even thinking. Instead, fix your attention on God. You'll be changed from the inside out. Readily recognize what he wants from you, and quickly respond to it. Unlike the culture around you, always dragging you down to its level of immaturity, God brings the best out of you, develops well-formed maturity in you.")

WEEDING OUT DECEPTION
(Recognizing the Truth)

⌇ Many keep their affairs restricted to their minds. But when they allow their minds to envision being involved in an affair or in other inappropriate activities or relationships, they are paving the way for their defenses to become so weakened that they eventually act out their thoughts. ⌇

4. Do you spend time imagining doing things you know are wrong? If so, what effect does it have on you?

5. Psalm 26:2 says, "Test me, O LORD, and try me, examine my heart and my mind." Are you, like David, *eager* for the Holy Spirit to examine your mind and test your thoughts? Why or why not?

⌇ Allowing your mind to be filled with images of sexually immoral or inappropriate behavior is like filling your mind with garbage. Garbage eventually rots, putrefying the soul and infecting your life and the lives of those you are closest to. One of the primary ways to avoid inappropriate fantasies and sexual misconduct is to resist such images and thoughts by limiting their access to your mind. This will require close monitoring of your reading, viewing, and listening habits, but once you make a habit of censorship, it will become second nature. 📖☕

6. Name the specific pieces of garbage you have allowed into your mind. What can you do to censor such garbage in the future?

📖 You stand before an important battle. You've decided that the slavery of sexual sin isn't worth your love of sexual sin. You're committed to removing every hint of it. But how? 📖

7. Do you really want to fight this battle, or does your love of sexual sin overpower your resolve? Be honest with yourself as you consider this question. Going to battle is tough; going to battle unprepared is foolish. Write your reflections here.

🐑 HARVESTING FULFILLMENT
(Applying the Truth)

🕮 Jesus wants us to love God *more* than any of the other things that demand our time and attention. We are to love God above anything else in this world, with as much strength and passion as each of us possibly can. We demonstrate this love for God by focusing our thoughts and energies on those things He's prepared for us to do and that are also pleasing to Him. God wants us to do just as Paul encouraged the people of Philippi to do: "Whatever is true, whatever is noble, whatever is right, whatever is pure, whatever is lovely, whatever is admirable—if anything is excellent or praiseworthy—think about such things" (Philippians 4:8). 🕮

8. Do you want to love God more than anything else? How would that look in your life if you pursued that desire?

9. What specific things do you feel God designed you to accomplish in life? What roles do you want to be fondly remembered for at the end of your life?

10. Ask God whether engaging in a healthy romantic relationship would drive you further from or closer to God's plan for your life. What are the pros and cons of being involved in a healthy romantic relationship?

11. Do the things you fill your mind with lead you *toward* God or *away* from God?

Be honest with yourself and with God. Only He knows what is best for you. Invite Him to shine His spotlight of truth into your heart and mind, showing you what you can do to make your mind more resistant even to being tempted in the first place.

In addition to screening what you allow into your mind, you can mentally rehearse righteous responses to temptations.

12. Have you ever rehearsed righteous responses to temptation? If so, what were they, and what was the result? If not, do you think it would strengthen you? Why or why not?

❧ GROWING TOGETHER
(Sharing the Truth in Small-Group Discussion)

13. What is the Bible's primary message about premarital sex? Back up everything you say with verses to be sure you are hearing God's instruction, not being swayed by cultural or even by Christian tradition.

📖 Reading or even studying the Bible won't keep you from sin. (Just look at all the pastors who are Bible scholars yet have engaged in sexual sin.) We have to *internalize* and *apply* what the Bible says. To renew the mind means to bring fresh, living thoughts into our minds in addition to keeping old, decaying thoughts at bay. 📖

14. Can you think of people who seem to know all the right answers, but don't live out what they say they believe? Do you ever feel like one of those people yourself? If so, how does it make you feel?

15. How do you get head knowledge to the heart? What role does the Holy Spirit play in this?

☕ You are a woman of conviction, and you live by those convictions. Others will see that your actions back up your words and that you give careful thought to the kind of woman you want to be. And if they ever come to realize that their lifestyles are not bringing them the fulfillment they long for, guess who they will likely run to for wise counsel? You guessed it: the woman who they know can teach them how to take every thought captive and live the overcoming life! ☕

16. Are you a woman of conviction? If so, what are your convictions or core beliefs on sex? How did you come by them? If you do not have strong convictions, are you ready to seek the Lord's desire for your life? How will you do that?

17. Do you have someone you could ask to help hold you accountable in your battle for sexual and emotional integrity? Are you willing to be held accountable in this area? Why or why not?

18. Are you able to extend grace to yourself when you fail to stand strong in your convictions? Do you believe God values you immeasurably even when you fail? How does this belief (or doubt) affect your life?

19. Are you able to extend grace to others when they fail or when they do not share your convictions? How do you balance grace and justice, truth and love?

20. Knowing that the battle for sexual integrity is tough, how can your words or actions help or hinder others in their own battles?

21. What kind of man do you think a woman of conviction would attract? Discuss how knowing ourselves and our moral standards affects our dating relationships.

Father God, thank You for creating women to have not only beautiful bodies, but strong minds. I offer my mind to You, Lord, and I pray that You will give me wisdom as I make decisions regarding my body. Help me always to remember that You are living in me and always renewing my mind. Amen.

guarding your heart

God told us to guard our hearts above all else—above our lives, our faith, our marriage, our pocketbook, our dreams, or whatever else we hold dear. In Proverbs He tells us: "Above all else, guard your heart, for it is the wellspring of life." (4:23). Why is it so important to God that we guard our hearts?

I believe the answer is in the word *wellspring,* which can also be interpreted as "source." The heart is the source of life. When God created us, He made our hearts central to our being—physically, spiritually, and emotionally.

Physically, the heart is at the center of your circulatory system. It pumps oxygenated blood throughout your body. If there is trouble inside your heart, your entire body is in danger of losing its life-giving flow of blood. Spiritually, your heart is the place where the Holy Spirit dwells when you invite Him into your life (see Ephesians 3:16-17). You receive salvation not just through head knowledge of God, but through belief in your heart that Jesus Christ is Lord (see Romans 10:9-10). Emotionally, your heart leaps for joy when you find delight in something or someone. It also aches when you experience disappointment with or loss of something or someone special.

The heart is literally and figuratively the core of all you are and all you experience in life, so when God says to guard it above all else, He is saying, "Protect the source of your life—the physical, spiritual, and emotional source of your well-being." Just as a lake will not be pure if its source is not pure, neither will our thoughts, words, and actions be pure if our hearts are not pure. Purity begins in our hearts. 📖🍵

📖 As the basis for your victory, did you know that God has provided you with everything you need for a life of purity? And it's better than a state-of-the-art global positioning system.

At Calvary, He purchased for you the freedom and authority to live in purity. That freedom and that authority are His gift to you through the presence of His Spirit, who took up residence within you when you gave your life to Christ. The freedom and authority are wrapped up in our new inner connection to His divine nature, which is the link that gives us His power and the fulfillment of His promises.... Regarding sexual purity, God knows the provision He's made for us. We aren't short on power or authority, but what we lack is *urgency*. We must choose to be strong and courageous to walk into purity. In the millisecond it takes to make that choice, the Holy Spirit will start guiding you and walking through the struggle with you. 📖

💧 PLANTING GOOD SEEDS
(Personally Seeking God's Truth)

To help you understand the pivotal role your heart plays in your sexual, emotional, and spiritual life, plant these good seeds in your heart:

> As water reflects a face,
>> so a [woman's] heart reflects the [woman]. (Proverbs 27:19)

I the LORD search the heart
and examine the mind,
to reward a [woman] according to [her] conduct,
according to what [her] deeds deserve. (Jeremiah 17:10)

1. According to these passages, why should you guard your heart?

As you seek to align your heart with God's plan for sexual and emotional integrity, plant this good seed in your heart:

You know the next commandment pretty well, too: "Don't go to bed with another's spouse." But don't think you've preserved your virtue simply by staying out of bed. Your *heart* can be corrupted by lust even quicker than your *body*. (Matthew 5:27-28, MSG)

2. What do you think Jesus was saying to His disciples in this passage? What does the passage say to you personally?

WEEDING OUT DECEPTION
(Recognizing the Truth)

While the need to love and to feel loved is a universal cry of the heart, the problem lies in where we look for this love. If we are not getting the love we need or want from a man—whether or not we have a husband—we may go searching for it. Some look in bars and others in business offices. Some look on college campuses and some look in churches. Some women look to male friends while others look to fantasy. When love eludes them, some women seek to medicate the pain of loneliness or rejection. Some take solace in food; others in sexual relationships with any willing partner. Some turn to soap operas; others to shopping; and still others to self-gratification.

If you have tried any of these avenues for long, you have likely come to a dead end. Your pursuit has left you longing for something greater, something deeper, something more.

3. Have you looked for love in problematic places? If so, where did you look, and what was the result?

4.   How have you sought to medicate the pain of loneliness or rejection? How has this worked for you in the short-term? in the long-term?

☙ Rather than running to the Ultimate Healer for relief from our emotional wounds, women often make idols of relationships—worshiping a man instead of God. We begin submitting to a man's and our own unholy desires rather than submitting to God's desires for our holiness and purity, thus becoming a slave to our passions.

When we peel back the layers of this issue, we can see the core problem: *doubt that God can truly satisfy our innermost needs.* So we look to a man who is not our husband and eventually discover that he doesn't "fix" us either. ☙

5.   Do you believe that at the core of sexual and emotional compromise is *doubt* that God is truly sufficient to satisfy our innermost needs? Explain your answer.

6. Do *you* doubt that God can meet *your* deepest needs? If so, write a prayer to God confessing this doubt and asking Him to remove it. If not, write a prayer affirming your belief that He is sufficient.

☏ [God] wants to dwell in every part of your heart, not just rent a room there. He wants to fill your heart to overflowing. Don't let guilt from past mistakes keep you from seeking this truly satisfying first-love relationship with Him. God does not despise you for the way you've tried to fill the void in your heart. He says, "Come now, let us reason together.... Though your sins are like scarlet, they shall be as white as snow; though they are red as crimson, they shall be like wool" (Isaiah 1:18). He is eager to cleanse your heart and teach you how to guard it from future pain and loneliness. ☏

7. What's the difference between having God dwell in your heart and just renting Him a room there? Has a guilty heart hindered you from experiencing the fullness of God's unconditional love for you? If so, how might you remedy that situation?

☕ **Attention** is based on what we see, whereas attraction is based on what we hear.... Maybe you've had the experience of noticing an incredibly handsome man, only to hear him open his mouth and yell at his kids, brag about his success, or complain about someone or something in a derogatory way....

He got your attention, but you felt no attraction. ☕

☕ In [the **attraction**] stage you become familiar enough with the person to know you are drawn to him, but you are not yet familiar enough to act affectionately toward that person.... Society has twisted our minds into thinking that if we are drawn to someone, we must want to have sex with him. But attraction isn't necessarily sexual. ☕

☕ When you know people well enough to discern that you are attracted to them, you might feel the urge to express your feelings by showing **affection** or displaying favor toward them. Signs of affection may be something tangible, such as a small gift or a kind note. ☕

☕ If you are single and hoping to develop a serious relationship with an interested, available man, **emotional arousal and attachment** is a natural, appropriate part of the courtship process. ☕

Red Light

Emotional Affairs
and Addictions

Yellow Light

Emotional Arousal
and Attachment

Affection

Green Light

Attraction

Attention

Identifying Green, Yellow, and
Red Levels of Emotional Connection

8. In your own words, explain the stages of the green-light level of emotional connection and why these are acceptable.

Attention

Attraction

9. In your own words, explain the stages of the yellow-light level of emotional connection and why we need to exercise caution with these stages.

Affection

Emotional Arousal and Attachment

10. Finally, explain the stages of the red-light level and why we need to stop before crossing these lines.

Emotional Affairs

Addictions

As you use caution and strive to refrain from red-light stages of emotional connection, you will regain the self-control, dignity, and self-respect you may have lost if you have compromised your sexual integrity. You can also expect a renewed…purity in your friendships or work relationships with…men. But best of all, when God looks on your pure heart and sees you are guarding it against unhealthy relationships, He will reward you with an even greater revelation of Himself.

11. What gives you the most incentive for avoiding the red-light stages of emotional connection? What specifically can you do to avoid crossing the line between integrity and compromise?

🐚 HARVESTING FULFILLMENT

(Applying the Truth)

📖 Holiness is not some nebulous thing. It's a series of right choices. You needn't wait for some holy cloud to form around you. You'll be holy when you choose not to sin. You're already free from the *power* of sexual immorality; you are not yet free from the *habit* of sexual immorality, until you choose to be—until you say, "That's enough! I'm choosing to live purely!" 📖

12. What impure habits will you choose to reject and eliminate from your life? What new, holy habits will you cultivate?

❧ GROWING TOGETHER

(Sharing the Truth in Small-Group Discussion)

📖 I encourage you to memorize the green-, yellow-, and red-light levels of emotional connection discussed in this chapter. Understanding exactly where the line is between emotional integrity and emotional compromise is one of the three keys to guarding your heart. The second key is being honest with yourself and learning to recognize any hidden motives, as this will tell you exactly where you stand in relationship to that line between integrity and compromise. The third key to guarding your heart (and the most important) is pursuing a first-love relationship with Jesus Christ. 📖

13. In your life, what guards have you set up to prevent yourself from crossing the line from integrity to compromise? How have they helped you?

14. Why is it important to guard your heart from emotional affairs?

15. Do you think we can ever become too preoccupied with guarding our hearts? Why or why not?

Consider this passage from *Every Woman's Battle,* then break into smaller groups and answer the following questions adapted from the close of chapter 6.

> ☕ While avoiding unhealthy emotional connections and relationships is important, it's not enough to guarantee success in keeping our hearts guarded against [emotional] compromise. The secret to ultimate emotional satisfaction is to pursue a mad, passionate love relationship with the One who made our hearts, the One who purifies our hearts, and the One who strengthens our hearts against worldly temptations. The secret is to focus your heart on your First Love. ☕

16. Have you *really* invested much time getting to know God personally and intimately? What have you done to get to know God?

17. Have you given God as many chances to satisfy your emotional needs as you've given other men? fantasy? Internet chat rooms?

18. Are you willing to make the choice to pray, to dance to worship music, or to go for a walk with God instead of picking up the phone to call a guy when you're lonely?

19. Are you willing to invite God to satisfy your every need by letting go of all the things, people, thoughts, and so on that you use to medicate your pain, fear, or loneliness, so that you might become totally dependent upon Him?

20. After answering these questions, can you honestly say that Jesus Christ is truly your first love? If not, what can you do to enhance the intimacy in your relationship with Him?

∞

Create in me a pure heart, O God, and renew a steadfast spirit within me. Do not cast me from your presence or take your Holy Spirit from me. Restore to me the joy of your salvation and grant me a willing spirit, to sustain me. Then I will teach transgressors your ways, and sinners will turn back to you. (PSALM 51:10-13)

being aware

 If we long to be women of sexual and emotional integrity, we must understand what a mighty weapon our words are. Words are what will lead us into an affair, or words will stop an affair before it ever begins.

I used to say, "I'm too weak to resist sexual temptation," and guess what? I was. But when God began dealing with me and sanctifying my mouth, I changed my tune. I started out by asking God, "Is it possible that sexual temptation could have no hold on me?" He gave me a glimmer of hope. Then I began claiming the statement, "Sexual temptation has no hold on me." After a while, I actually began believing it wholeheartedly. Now I can honestly declare with conviction, "Sexual temptation has no hold on me!"

If we tell ourselves that we can't resist sexual or emotional temptation, we will likely fall into temptation. But if we tell ourselves that we will not give in to sexual and emotional temptation, then we will be far more likely to back up our words with corresponding actions. That is how you become a woman of integrity—a person whose lip lines up with her life and vice versa.

📖 Before we started winning our own battles for purity, we had a number of false starts—partly because we hadn't really made a decision. We sort of wanted purity, and sort of didn't. We didn't understand the enemy and how to approach it. The whole business of sexual integrity was mysterious.... Now that we've touched on Satan's part in our battle against impurity, let's focus on whether sexual impurity represents some form of demon possession.

You aren't possessed by the devil when impurity runs rampant in your life, and you don't need an exorcism. Although it sometimes *feels* like an evil gremlin inside you is driving you to sin, these are merely the compulsions of your bad habits and hormones. You're simply out of control and must bring them all back under the control of your regenerated spirit....

While there may not be spiritual oppression involved in your battle, there'll always be spiritual *opposition*. The enemy is constantly near your ear. He doesn't want you to win this fight, and he knows the lies that so often break men's confidence and their will to win. Expect to hear lies and plenty of them.

What we've told you is the truth. There *is* peace and tranquillity for you on the other side of this war. There *is* immeasurable spiritual gain. 📖

🪣 PLANTING GOOD SEEDS
(Personally Seeking God's Truth)

As you consider the effect of your words on your relationship with God, others, and yourself, plant these good seeds in your heart:

> If anyone considers [herself] religious and yet does not keep a tight rein on [her] tongue, [she] deceives [herself] and [her] religion is worthless. (James 1:26)

The tongue is a small part of the body, but it makes great boasts. Consider what a great forest is set on fire by a small spark. The tongue also is a fire, a world of evil among the parts of the body. It corrupts the whole person, sets the whole course of his life on fire. (James 3:5-6)

1. How has your tongue helped or hurt your relationship with God? others? yourself?

As you seek to integrate your words with your life of sexual and emotional integrity, plant these seeds in your heart:

For out of the overflow of the heart the mouth speaks. The good [woman] brings good things out of the good stored up in [her], and the evil [woman] brings evil things out of the evil stored up in [her]. But I tell you that [women] will have to give account on the day of judgment for every careless word they have spoken. For by your words you will be acquitted, and by your words you will be condemned. (Matthew 12:34-37)

But among you there must not be even a hint of sexual immorality, or of any kind of impurity…because these are improper for God's holy people. Nor should there be obscenity, foolish talk or coarse joking, which are out of place, but rather thanksgiving. (Ephesians 5:3-4)

2.   What needs to change first: your heart or your words? Explain your answer.

⚒ WEEDING OUT DECEPTION
(Recognizing the Truth)

🍵 While many women flirt with men intentionally, others don't realize that their amorous comments are inappropriate. We hear this kind of language so often in the media that flirting can be a natural or automatic response. Some women are too naive to recognize the impact that their words and mannerisms have on the opposite sex. Other women are well aware, but are so hungry for affirmation that they continue to jeopardize their integrity in order to fish for compliments anyway. 🍵

3.   Are you aware of the impact your words and actions have on men? If so, how do you use that knowledge? If not, how will you learn to be more aware?

4. If you enjoy flirting with men, what do you think you might be looking to gain? Has flirting ever put you in an uncomfortable or compromising situation? Explain your answer.

☕ Women can be far too nurturing in situations, even when red flags begin to surface. We often think, *But he needs me... I'm just trying to be a friend... How can I possibly* not *help? That would not be very Christianlike!* ☕

5. Do you tend to be overly nurturing with men, frequently playing the "mother" or "counselor" or "best friend" role? If so, what may be behind this tendency?

6. Have you experienced temptations to compromise your sexual and emotional integrity because you were being "too kind for your own good"? If so, how can you overcome this tendency?

◈ While the Bible doesn't specifically state how long a skirt should be or what sections of skin should always be covered, we can always go back to Jesus's commandment as a guideline for how we are to dress: love your neighbor as yourself. ◈

7. Are you prone to dress for attention rather than for respect? What effect do you think your appearance has on men? How do you think your dress affects their opinion of you?

8. Are you more concerned with inner beauty or with outer beauty? How does that prioritizing affect your life?

❧ HARVESTING FULFILLMENT
(Applying the Truth)

◈ In our quest for relational intimacy, remember there is Someone we can whisper our hearts' desires to and get our boosts from who isn't going to jeopardize our integrity but will strengthen it.

If you are thinking, *No way will talking to God ever excite me like talking to a man,* then you haven't allowed yourself to be courted by our Creator. The same God whose words possessed the power to form the entire universe longs to whisper into your hungry heart words that have the power to thrill you, heal you, and draw you into a deeper love relationship than you ever imagined possible. A guy may say that you look fine, but God's Word says, "The king is enthralled by your beauty" (Psalm 45:11). A man may tell you, "Of course I love you," but God says, "I have loved you with an everlasting love; I have drawn you with loving-kindness" (Jeremiah 31:3). Even your husband may tell you, "I'm committed to you until death," but God says, "Never will I leave you; never will I forsake you" (Hebrews 13:5).

9. Do you believe that God can love you more than a man can? How does that make you feel?

10. What exactly are you longing for that a romantic relationship offers? Do you believe that a relationship with God will offer all that and more? Why or why not?

11. If you find fulfillment in God, does that mean you cannot also desire a relationship with a man? What is the relationship of one to the other?

12. In what ways can deep friendships with other women meet some of our longings for connection? In what ways do they fall short?

❧ GROWING TOGETHER
(Sharing the Truth in Small-Group Discussion)

📖 Picture this scenario: You know that your neighbor is dieting to lose ten pounds before her wedding. You also know that if she does not lose the weight, her dress will be too tight and she will feel uncomfortable on her big day. But you are a gourmet dessert chef and you crave the affirmation that you are a good cook, so you insist that your neighbor eat the pound cake and fudge and coconut cream pie samples that you bring over to her house every day. Are you acting lovingly or selfishly toward your neighbor?

Now consider this: You know that men are visually stimulated at the sight of a woman's body, especially a scantily clad body. You are also aware that godly men are trying desperately to honor their wives by not allowing their eyes to stray. In light of this, if you insist on wearing clothes that reveal your sleek curves and tanned skin, are you acting lovingly or selfishly? This is a good thing to ask yourself each morning as you are getting dressed for the day. Rather than asking, "What man will I come across today and will this catch his eye?" try asking, "Would wearing this outfit be a loving expression, not causing my brothers to stumble and fall?" 🍵

13. Do you think it is your responsibility to dress modestly for the sake of men who struggle with lust? Why or why not?

🍵 While it may be okay to act amorously (as if desiring romance) toward someone you are interested in developing a mutually beneficial relationship with, flirting is a different matter. Flirting could also be called "teasing," as the person doing the flirting has no serious intent. Regardless of her marital status, should a woman stir up a man (emotionally or physically) when she has no intention of pursuing a relationship with him? Is it loving to tease someone with your attentions and affections if you have no desire to fulfill any hopes you may arouse? In my opinion, showing a sincere love and respect for others allows no room for flirting or teasing. 🍵

14. What is it that makes flirting so much fun? Do you think it is okay for a single woman to flirt with a man if she has no intention of investing in a healthy romantic relationship? Explain your answer.

☕ It has been said that men use conversation as a means of communicating information, but women use conversation as a means of bonding. While communicating and bonding with our…children or female friends is great, communicating and bonding…with men we wouldn't choose to date is dangerous and often destructive. And yes, the more we communicate with a person, the more we bond, so we would do well to take a lesson from the men in this area and learn to stick to business a little better. We can learn to communicate with men in friendly but to-the-point ways that will not jeopardize our emotional integrity. ☕

15. Have you ever bonded with a man unintentionally due to excess communication? What did you learn from this experience?

16. What boundaries have you implemented (or may need to implement) to keep from bonding with men in inappropriate ways, whether in person, over the phone, or in cyberspace?

17. Why do you think women find it so appealing to comfort men? What do you think it is that they are really seeking? When is this kind of connection inappropriate, and when is it permissible?

18. Do you believe that resisting an emotional or sexual affair may be as easy as choosing appropriate words and avoiding inappropriate words in your conversations with men? Why or why not?

☕ Make time to retreat to a quiet place with the Lover of your soul. Speak whatever is on your heart, and then *listen* as God speaks straight from His heart directly to yours. ☕

19. Have you ever tried to listen to what God has to say to you? If so, what was the result? If not, what is keeping you from doing that?

20. What does "Lover of your soul" mean to you? Have you ever experienced unconditional love?

Dear Jesus, I am overwhelmed with gratefulness as I think about how much You love me. I want so much to become the precious woman that You know me to be, that You created me to be. Help me to see clearly how You would have me live so that I can bring joy to You and to me. Amen.

surrendering

If you want to win the battle for sexual integrity, you must let go of past emotional pain. Maybe a father who was absent, either emotionally or physically, wounded you. Maybe the distance in your relationship with your mother left you feeling desperately lonely. Perhaps your siblings or friends never treated you with dignity or respect. If you were abused in any way (physically, sexually, or verbally) as a child, maybe you have anger and pain that has yet to be reconciled.

Perhaps old lovers took advantage of your vulnerabilities, strung you along, or were unfaithful to you. Or maybe you've never understood why God allowed _____ to happen (you fill in the blank). Regardless of its source, we must surrender the pain from our past in order to stand strong in the battle for sexual and emotional integrity.

Satan fights you with lies, while your body fights you with the desires and strength of deeply entrenched bad habits. To win [the battle for purity], you need a sword and a shield. Of all the parts of your battle plan, this is likely the most important.

You'll need a good Bible verse to use as a sword and rallying point.

Just one? It may be useful to memorize several verses of Scripture about purity, as they work to eventually transform and wash the mind. But in the cold-turkey, day-to-day fight against impurity, having several memory verses might be as cumbersome as strapping on a hundred-pound backpack to engage in hand-to-hand combat. You aren't agile enough.

That's why we recommend a single "attack verse," and it better be quick. [For men,] we suggest the opening line of Job 31: "I made a covenant with my eyes."…

Your shield—a protective verse that you can reflect on and draw strength from even when you aren't in the direct heat of battle—may be even more important than your sword, because it places temptation out of earshot.

We suggest selecting this verse as your shield: "Flee from sexual immorality…. You are not your own; you were bought at a price. Therefore honor God with your body" (1 Corinthians 6:18-20). 📖

🪴 PLANTING GOOD SEEDS
(Personally Seeking God's Truth)

To help you let go of past emotional pain and seek to reconcile relationships, plant this good seed in your heart:

> Bear with each other and forgive whatever grievances you may have against one another. Forgive as the Lord forgave you. (Colossians 3:13)

1. Have you forgiven the people who have hurt you? If so, what has been the result in your life? If not, what is keeping you from doing that? (Keep in mind that forgiveness is simply letting go of your right to seek vengeance; it is not excusing the behavior.)

2. Have you received the forgiveness the Lord has offered you? If so, what has been the result in your life? If not, what is keeping you from doing that?

As you recognize that nothing short of God's grace will help you overcome sexual temptations, plant this good seed in your heart:

> For the grace of God that brings salvation has appeared to all [women]. It teaches us to say "No" to ungodliness and worldly passions, and to live self-controlled, upright and godly lives in this present age, while we wait for the blessed hope—the glorious appearing of our great God and Savior, Jesus Christ, who gave himself for us to redeem us from all wickedness and to purify for himself a people that are his very own, eager to do what is good. (Titus 2:11-14)

3. Are you eager to live a self-controlled, upright, and godly life? How does knowing that God's grace to resist sexual sin is available to anyone who believes in Christ affect your battle plan?

✎ WEEDING OUT DECEPTION
(Recognizing the Truth)

4. Use the chart on the next page to process some of the past emotional pain you have experienced that has possibly left you vulnerable to sexual and/or emotional compromise. If you have more than one relationship to reconcile in this way, you may reproduce this chart.

To enter the process of forgiveness, you must take these steps:
- Acknowledge your anger and hurt. It is very real and God knows it is there.
- Realize that holding on to this pain only holds you back.
- Consciously let go of any need for revenge.
- Consider the source of your pain: hurting people hurt other people. Put yourself in their shoes.

Who is the person who caused my past emotional pain? How?	
How did this make me feel?	
How did this event/relationship make me vulnerable to temptation?	
How does this still affect me?	
What personal pain may have caused this person to hurt me?	
How does my unforgiveness affect this person?	
How does my unforgiveness affect me and my loved ones?	
How would my forgiveness affect this person?	
How would my forgiveness affect me and my loved ones?	
Can I cancel this debt as Jesus canceled mine? Why or why not?	
How can I pray for this person?	
How can I avoid causing this same pain in others' lives?	

- Pray earnestly for those who hurt you, asking God to heal the wounds that cause them to wound others.
- Pray that your wounds do not cause you to do the same to others. ☕

5. Have you genuinely acknowledged your anger and pain? Why or why not? What has been the result?

6. Do you believe that God knows your pain? How does this belief (or doubt) affect your life?

☕ Our heavenly Father…never *forces* us to take His hand but allows us to experience the need for His hand so that we will *desire* it. When we tell ourselves, *I can handle this battle on my own, I don't need help, I can manage without accountability,* we set ourselves up for a fall.

I recently heard a statement that made my heart skip a beat: "You are never more like Satan than when you are full of pride." Isn't it true? Pride got Satan expelled from heaven. Pride hinders sinners from asking Jesus to be their Savior and submitting to His Lordship. And pride keeps Christians from repenting from the things that cause them to stumble and fall, such as sexual and emotional compromise. ☕

7. Have you been aware that God is extending His hand of help to you? How have you responded?

8. Do you struggle with pride? To better discern whether or not you do, take a few moments to define pride for yourself and name its symptoms. What can you do to prevent pride from coming into your heart (or to remove it)?

☕ Perhaps you are wondering if you even *want* to cut some habits out altogether. Maybe you really *like* doing what you are doing or thinking what you are thinking.

One of the most honest prayers I've ever heard is, "Lord, forgive me for the sins that I enjoy!" Sin often feels good (at least initially), or else it wouldn't be tempting. But recognizing how your pet sins ultimately impact your life may inspire you to surrender them. ☕

9. Do you have any sins that you find yourself wanting to hold on to? Take a moment to imagine what your life would look like with that habit completely gone from your life, desires, and actions. Which scenario do you prefer (as it is now, or as it could be)? Why?

HARVESTING FULFILLMENT
(Applying the Truth)

Why is [fear] such a hindrance? Because *fear* is the opposite of *faith*.... How can we focus on what we know God will do when we think we are doomed? Such lack of faith says to God, "Even though you've carried me this far, you are probably going to fail me now, aren't you?"...

The same is true in our battle against sexual and emotional compromise. Many women are steeped in the fear of being alone, the fear of not being taken care of, the fear of not having another man on the hook in case the current one gets away. We can be so afraid of compromising tomorrow that we fail to take notice and celebrate the fact that we are standing firm today.

10. On a scale of one to ten, how strong is your desire to be taken care of? Do you believe your desire for a relationship with a man is healthy or not?

11.   How does your attitude affect your actions in regard to men? How can you give all your fears over to God today?

12.   Why do you think some women fear genuine intimacy (such as revealing our innermost thoughts to those we love or to God) yet crave superficial intimacy (such as a rendezvous with an attractive stranger)?

13.   How can we cultivate the courage to engage fully in genuine intimacy with one man and with God rather than seeking escape routes (fantasy, emotional affairs, and so on)?

The white flag you will be waving as you surrender your past pain, present pride, and future fear is *not* a symbol of defeat. It is a symbol of victory, for it represents purity. You will be washed clean of all compromise as you allow God to transform you—heart and mind—into a woman who forgives her debtors, walks in humility, and faces the future with confidence in her Creator and Sustainer. 📖☕

14. Do you believe that surrendering your fears to God is a sign of strength or weakness? Explain your answer in the context of your life experiences.

🍃 GROWING TOGETHER
(Sharing the Truth in Small-Group Discussion)

📖☕ One day as I was beating myself up for yet another emotional affair, my best friend interrupted me with these sobering words: "Do you know what you are saying about the blood that Jesus shed for you when you refuse to forgive yourself for your past? You are saying that His blood wasn't good enough for you. It didn't have enough power to cleanse you." She was right. Underlying all of my self-pity was the belief that what Jesus did for me couldn't possibly be enough to rid me of my stain. I needed some special miracle to set me free, and until I got that miracle, I had to beat myself up as an act of penance. 📖☕

15. Why do you think it is much harder to forgive ourselves for mistakes in judgment than to forgive others?

16. Do you most need to personally surrender past emotional pain, present pride, or future fear? Explain.

17. What victory is gained as a result of this surrender? How will you be affected by this victory? How does that make you feel and why?

📖 Keep your eyes open for that accountability partner. Perhaps it will be a friend or a sister, a teacher, a counselor, or a mentor. While you may be tempted to look for someone who can sympathize with you, you may have more long-term success with someone who isn't struggling herself or who has already overcome such a struggle. Hitching two weak oxen together to plow a field is not nearly as effective as hitching a weak ox with a strong one.

When you have a mentor who can show you how to thrive on a diet of humility, you may discover a healing change in your appetite. Remember, we cannot sin and win. If there is sexual or emotional sin in your life, you must starve it to death. You can't just "trim it down" or it will just grow right back, even larger than before. Sin must be cut out completely. 📖

18. Have you found this group to provide good accountability relationships? If so, how has that helped you? If not, what do you think is hindering that?

19. Have you been able to starve the sexual and emotional sins in your life? If so, what has been the result? If not, what do you think will help you to do that?

20. Do you sometimes lose hope that you will ever change? How does this affect your battle against sexual immorality? How do you regain your hope?

21. Do you remember when you first became aware of the sacrifice Jesus made for you? Take a few moments to relive that time in your life so that you can revive your awe of God's gift to you. Encourage others with your reflection.

Lord, thank You for showing us that the way to victory is through surrendering our past emotional pain, our present prideful sins, and our future fear. Help us to let go of the things that hinder our spiritual growth and make us vulnerable to temptation. Free us to enjoy the sexual and emotional fulfillment that You desire for us to experience. In the name of Jesus. Amen.

cultivating true intimacy

Both men and women have handled counterfeit intimacy for so long that they've lowered their standards and settled for far less than the real thing. Men look for satisfaction through sex, but physical intimacy alone doesn't bring ultimate fulfillment. Many women can attest to the fact that just because a man is fantastic in bed doesn't mean he fulfills her emotionally. Even great sex in marriage is not the same as genuine intimacy....

Genuine sexual intimacy involves all components of our sexuality—the physical, mental, emotional, and spiritual. When these four are combined, the result is an elixir that stirs the soul, heals the heart, boggles the mind, and genuinely satisfies.

How unfortunate are those who have never tasted the sweetness of sexual intimacy as God intended it to be because they have accepted one or two parts as a counterfeit for the whole....

When you first picked up this book subtitled *Discovering God's Plan for Sexual and Emotional Fulfillment,* perhaps you thought it was going to be all about how to have great sex. Well it is, but probably not the kind you were expecting. I hope that you've been pleasantly surprised as you learned about the things holding you back from true sexual intimacy.

📖 But your mind is orderly, and your worldview colors what comes through it. The mind will allow these impure thoughts only if they "fit" the way you look at the world. As you set up the perimeter of defense for your mind, your brain's worldview will be transformed by a new matrix of allowed thoughts, or "allowables."

Within the old matrix of your thinking, lust fit perfectly and in that sense was "orderly." But with a new, purer matrix firmly in place, lustful thoughts will bring disorder. Your brain, acting as a responsible policeman, nabs these lustful thoughts even before they rise to consciousness. Essentially the brain begins cleaning itself, so elusive enemies like double entendres and daydreams, which are hard to control on the conscious level, simply vanish on their own.

This transformation of the mind takes some time as you wait for the old sexual pollution to be washed away. It's much like living near a creek that becomes polluted when a sewer main breaks upstream. After repair crews replace the cracked sewage pipe, it will still take some time for the water downstream to clear.

In transforming your mind, you'll be taking an active, conscious role in capturing rogue thoughts, but in the long run, the mind will wash itself and will begin to work naturally for you and your purity by capturing such thoughts. With the eyes bouncing away from sexual images and the mind policing itself, your defenses will grow incredibly strong. 📖

🖋 PLANTING GOOD SEEDS
(Personally Seeking God's Truth)

As you seek to establish a new way of viewing sexuality, plant this good seed in your heart:

Do not conform any longer to the pattern of this world, but be transformed by the renewing of your mind. Then you will be able to test and approve what God's will is—his good, pleasing and perfect will. (Romans 12:2)

1. When you think about your sin, you may decide to change your behavior, but will you make the commitment to change the way you think? How will doing so help you in your battle against sexual impurity?

2. When your friends or acquaintances or TV characters live life in a way that seems appealing but wrong to you, do you have a difficult time rejecting that behavior for yourself? What would be the best thing for you to do in order to avoid falling into that sin?

As you learn to cultivate holy thinking, plant the good seed of James 5:16 in your heart:

Therefore confess your sins to each other and pray for each other so that you may be healed.

3. How does confessing your sins and praying for others bring about the renewal of your mind? Can you think of someone who would be a good prayer partner for you?

WEEDING OUT DECEPTION
(Recognizing the Truth)

Imagine wanting to give a squirrel a nut. How would you do it? Would you chase the squirrel around the yard, grab him by his scrawny neck, and force the nut into his chubby cheeks? Of course not. You cannot require a squirrel to take a nut from you. However, you can inspire the squirrel to do this by simply placing a nut in your open palm, lying down beneath a tree, and falling asleep. When it's the squirrel's idea to take the nut, he'll do it. Communicating intimately with [others] is very similar to giving a squirrel a nut. Requiring it is futile. Intimacy can, however, be inspired.

4. Have you attempted to force the issue of intimacy with others? How, specifically, have you done this? Has it worked for you? Why or why not?

5. When you seek out intimacy, are you equally concerned for the other person's fulfillment as you are for your own? Why or why not? If you do consider the other person's fulfillment, how does this transform your understanding of intimacy?

🕮 As we learn to speak each other's love language, our love tanks are filled and we protect our…relationships from outside physical or emotional temptations. When either or both partners fail to recognize and meet the needs of their mate, these temptations can become overwhelming. I frequently hear women say (and have said it myself), "I'm so tempted because he doesn't meet my emotional needs!" But before you take aim at [others] for not meeting your emotional needs, look into your own emotional mirror. 🕮

6. Do you know exactly what your emotional needs are? Do you know your own love language? Why is it important to understand this about yourself?

📖 What happens if we don't starve the attractions? What if we play with the attractions a little? Won't the passage of time kill the attractions anyway?

Most of the time, yes, but you can't take a chance. An improper relationship is not pleasing to God, no matter how "innocent" it appears.

In summary, you have a mind that runs where it wills. It must be tamed. Our best tactic is to starve the attractions, limiting the generation of impure thoughts and the damage they bring to our...relationship[s]. 📖

7. Do you find yourself feeding your sinful desires? What do you think would happen if you attempted to starve those desires? Does that choice sound healthy or unhealthy to you? Why?

8. Do you believe you are immune to a sexual or emotional affair? Does that cause you to keep your guard up or down?

9. Have you ever found an "innocent" attraction taking a wrong turn? If so, what would have happened if you had been guarding yourself? If not, how do you think you avoided the situation?

📖 HARVESTING FULFILLMENT
(Applying the Truth)

📖 In *The Final Quest,* Rick Joyner writes, "Spiritual maturity is always dictated by our willingness to sacrifice our own desires for the desires of others or for the interests of the kingdom."

Purifying your eyes and mind is more than a command—it's also a sacrifice. And as you make that sacrifice, as you lay down your desires, blessings will flow. Your spiritual life will experience new joy and power, and your [relationships] will blossom. 📖

10. How might sacrificing yourself for the benefit of others or for the interests of the kingdom ultimately bring you great reward? Have you experienced this in your life? Explain.

11. Have you been able to master guarding your eyes and mind in the battle against sexual impurity? If so, what has helped you find success? If not, try thinking of letting go of your own desires as a gift to other people—and enjoy the process of blessing others. If you did this, what do you expect would be the result in your life?

❧ GROWING TOGETHER
(Sharing the Truth in Small-Group Discussion)

12. Considering what you have studied in this book, what type of "intimacy busters"—roadblocks to an intimate relationship with God or your future spouse—have you struggled with in the past?

13. How have you overcome those issues, and what advice do you have for others currently struggling in those areas?

14. Which "intimacy boosters"—beneficial actions to improve your relationship with God or your future spouse—have you discovered to be helpful? What effect have they had on your ultimate fulfillment? on your dating relationships?

15. Often single women feel pressured into pursuing a marriage relationship because they believe sex in marriage to be far more fulfilling than anything they could experience (including intimacy with Christ) as a single person. Do you feel this pressure? What can you do to find fulfillment as a single person?

16. Many singles, including Christian singles, engage in sexual activity. Do you believe it is possible for them to experience lovemaking as the act of worship God designed it to be? Why or why not?

📖 You may think affairs…happen so infrequently that you can confidently say, "Well, *I* would never do such a thing!" But words like that mean nothing if you have any sense. We urge you: Please, protect yourself. Don't be defenseless because you *can* get fooled. 📖

17.   Why do you think Christians so often think themselves immune to affairs? What defenses have you set up for yourself?

Father, thank You for creating me to be a beautiful woman, physically, emotionally, mentally, and spiritually. I pray that Your plan will be made perfect in my life. In Jesus's name. Amen.

retreating with the Lord

A radiant bride greeted her guests with a brilliant smile as she entered the reception hall after the wedding ceremony. She gracefully moved and milled about the room, the train of her stunning white gown flowing along the floor behind her, her veil cascading down her button-adorned back.

She conversed with each guest one by one, taking the time to mingle and soak up the compliments. "You look absolutely lovely." "Your dress is divine." "I've never seen a more beautiful bride." "What a stunning ceremony." The lavish praises rang on and on. The bride couldn't be more proud or more appreciative of the crowd's adoration. She could have listened to them swoon over her all evening. As a matter of fact, she did.

But where was the groom? All the attention focused on the bride and never once did she call anyone's attention to her husband. She didn't even notice his absence at her side. Scanning the room, I searched for him, wondering, "Where could he be?"

I finally found him, but not where I expected him to be. The groom stood alone over in the corner of the room with his head down. As he stared at his ring, twisting the gold band that had just been placed on his finger by his bride, tears trickled down his cheeks and onto his hands. That is when I noticed the nail scars. The groom was Jesus.

He waited, but the bride never once turned her face toward her groom. She never held His hand. She never introduced the guests to Him. She operated independently of Him.

I awoke from my dream with a sick feeling in my stomach. "Lord, is this how I made you feel when I was looking for love in all the wrong places?" I wept at the thought of hurting Him so deeply.

Unfortunately, this dream illustrates exactly what is happening between God and millions of His people. He betroths Himself to us, we take His name (as "Christians"), and then we go about our lives looking for love, attention, and affection from every source under the sun except from the Son of God, the Lover of our souls.

Oh, how Jesus longs for His own to acknowledge Him, to introduce Him to our friends, to withdraw to be alone with Him, to cling to Him for our identity, to gaze longingly into His eyes, to love Him with all our heart and soul.

What about you? Do you have this kind of love relationship with Christ? Do you experience the inexplicable joy of intimacy with the One who loves you with a passion far deeper, far greater than anything you could find here on earth? I know from experience that you can. 📖

📖 If Christians were consumed by God's purposes, it would first be reflected in our marriages. But the rates of divorce, adultery, and marital dissatisfaction in the Christian church reveal our hearts.... [Someday you may find] it difficult to cherish your one and only. We understand that sentiment. To cherish means to treat with tenderness and to hold dear, and you want to feel the romantic urge to do those things. But what if you don't feel like it? Something with such ramifications upon your sexual purity...cannot be left to feelings alone. 📖

🌱 PLANTING GOOD SEEDS
(Personally Seeking God's Truth)

As you cultivate a more intimate friendship with God, plant the good seed of Proverbs 22:11 in your heart:

> [She] who loves a pure heart and whose speech is gracious will have the king for [her] friend.

1. On a scale of one to ten, how intimate do you feel your friendship with the Lord is? How does the level of your relationship with Him affect your relationships with others?

2. Your speech cannot be gracious if your heart is not pure before God. How do you make your heart pure?

As you seek to embrace the magnitude of God's faithfulness, righteousness, and lavish love for you, plant these good seeds in your heart:

I am my beloved's and my beloved is mine.
>   (Song of Solomon 6:3, RSV)

I will betroth you to me forever;
>   I will betroth you in righteousness and justice,
>   in love and compassion.
I will betroth you in faithfulness,
>   and you will acknowledge the LORD. (Hosea 2:19-20)

Your love, O LORD, reaches to the heavens,
>   your faithfulness to the skies.
Your righteousness is like the mighty mountains,
>   your justice like the great deep....
>   How priceless is your unfailing love!
Both high and low among [women]
>   find refuge in the shadow of your wings.
They feast on the abundance of your house;
>   you give them drink from your river of delights. (Psalm 36:5-8)

3. Are you feasting on the abundance of God's house and drinking from His river of delights? How did you get to that place? Or are you starving spiritually, wondering why you are unfulfilled in your relationships? How might you change that situation and feeling?

WEEDING OUT DECEPTION
(Recognizing the Truth)

Maybe you are wondering how to get from where you are now to this much deeper, more gratifying level of intimacy with Jesus Christ. It would help to look at where our spiritual journey begins as believers and how our relationship with God evolves as we travel down the path toward spiritual maturity. Life coach and international lecturer Jack Hill (www.royal-quest .com) explains that there are six progressive levels of relationship with God, as found in the following metaphors in Scripture:

- potter/clay relationship
- shepherd/sheep relationship
- master/servant relationship
- friend/friend relationship
- father/daughter relationship
- groom/bride relationship

I believe God gave us these metaphors to increase our understanding of His many-faceted personality and to help us comprehend the depth of His perfect love for us (although the human mind cannot fathom such depth). These metaphors illustrate the maturing of our love relationship with God. Just as children develop physically until they reach adulthood, believers in Christ develop spiritually in stages as we walk down the road to spiritual maturity. As we examine the dynamics of each of these stages, perhaps you can discern what level of intimacy you are currently experiencing in your walk with God. You can also determine what level of connection you can anticipate as your relationship with God continues to blossom.

4. Which of the above metaphors best describes your relationship with God? Explain. What level of intimacy with God do you wish to have with Him?

5. Do you allow God to shape your life continually so it always brings Him honor? If so, how do you do that? If not, what would it look like to do so?

6. Do you trust Him as your guide and follow Him? How have your past experiences affected your trust of God?

7. Do you more often obey or disobey God? Do you struggle with authority figures? How do you balance self-respect with genuine humility before God?

8. Do you spend time reading the Bible so that you can have a better understanding of God's will? Do you confide your struggles and joys to the Lord? Would you consider that kind of relating a friendship? Why or why not?

9. Do you tend to "perform" with God, or have you learned to accept His unconditional love? How do you live out your faith without trying to work for your salvation?

HARVESTING FULFILLMENT
(Applying the Truth)

📖 I have found that God's affirmation fills my emotional tank even more than any human's flattering words will. When I sense the God of the universe saying to me, "I see everything you are doing and your hard work brings me great joy.... You are so beautiful to me even when you are sleeping.... I see your heart and you are so very special to me," His sentiments send me reeling further than any man ever could. 📖

10. How do you feel when you consider that God loves you intimately, as His spiritual bride? How can you respond to Him, considering Him to be a faithful husband?

11. If you are not currently at the level of relationship with God that you desire to be, what activities can you incorporate into your life in order to cultivate such intimacy? Are there others that you can add to this list (abbreviated from chapter 11 of *Every Woman's Battle*)?

    ____ a date night with Jesus
    ____ walking and talking with the Lord
    ____ a restful rendezvous with God
    ____ retreating with the Lord
    ____ other _____
    ____ other _____

In addition to putting aside some time each day to rest in the arms of God and converse with Jesus, I recommend that you schedule a sabbatical alone with God at least once or twice each year. Based on the word *sabbath,* a sabbatical is an extended amount of time set apart for the further cultivation of a love relationship with Jesus.

12. If a retreat with the Lord sounds inviting to you, circle the idea(s) that appeal to you most:

"Past, Present, and Future" Retreat—releasing past wounds through letters of forgiveness, examining present priorities, and evaluating future spiritual, relational, professional, financial, or physical goals.

Hobby Retreat—doing what you enjoy doing most (painting, reading, writing, and so on) while enjoying time alone with the Lord.

"Prayer, Praise, and Pampering" Retreat—giving yourself a spiritual spa treatment in preparation to enter His throne room in worship.

Intercessor's Retreat—praying for those God has laid on your heart and writing notes of encouragement.

"Thanks for the Memories" Retreat—updating your photo albums and giving thanks for all of the special friends and family who adorn the pages.

"Leaving a Legacy of Love" Retreat—reflecting on the spiritual markers of your life and communicating those in a special letter to your children (or other loved ones).

Other

_____

_____

🍃 GROWING TOGETHER
(Sharing the Truth in Small-Group Discussion)

> 🍵 Response time is a vital part of my prayer life. [God] already knows what is on my heart without my saying a word. I need to make time to listen to what is on His heart because without listening I'll never have a clue. 🍵

13. What percentage of your prayer time is spent talking to God, and what percentage is spent listening? If the same percentages were applied to an earthly friendship, what would the result be? Would there be mutual intimacy, or would the relationship feel one-sided?

14. Do you have a specific place, time of day, or activity that you engage in where you feel especially connected to God? If so, share that with the group.

15. If God spoke to you (or the entire group) right now, what do you think He would say? How would He say it? How would you respond?

📖 God never forgot what we often forget—namely, the curse of Eden is a grinding curse. Life is a steamroller, making pancakes of conditions and easily mashing the naive contracts we create. In our dreams for marriage, maybe we forget that we would still have to work long hours by the sweat of our brow to eat, and that we wouldn't always see each other as much as we wish. Maybe we forget that we will sometimes be beaten up and used by bosses, our minds so numb we just don't want to talk when we get home. Maybe we forget that with the pain in childbirth comes bodies that never regain their former shape.

Any number of trials and tribulations might make conditions impossible to meet, but we demanded guarantees anyway, demanding some form of Eden from our [relationships], when all the time our place is to cherish [each other] unconditionally.

That doesn't sound much like Eden to us. We don't like our place. So our inner defenses are let down, and we lose our concern for God's purposes. 📖

16. When you began this study, were you hoping to have all your problems solved? How does it feel to realize that there will always be problems? How can you embrace hope while you are living in an imperfect world?

17. Now that this study is drawing to a close, what steps will you take to continue to guard your mind and heart so that you will be able to maintain sexual and emotional integrity?

I'm also not promising that God will heal you the same way that He healed me. Healing comes gradually for most women, but God knows the process that will work best for you. He alone knows how to deliver you out of the chaos of compromise into a place of victory.

While I hope you use this book and its accompanying workbook to guide you to a place of mental, emotional, spiritual, and physical integrity, I encourage you all the more to look directly to God to guide you there. He knows the way. Simply rendezvous with Him regularly for direction.

18. Have you been envious when you've seen growth in others or prideful when you've seen your own growth? If so, how can you overcome these feelings?

19. How exactly have you seen God work in your life over these past eight or twelve weeks?

20. List several words or phrases that describe how you feel about what you've accomplished while using this workbook.

Lord Jesus, the thing I long for more than anything else is to grow closer to You. I know that nothing else will matter unless I have received the relationship You so graciously offer me. Help me to embrace my role as Your intimate friend, Your precious child, and Your chosen bride. Draw me into Your presence each day and fill me to overflowing with Your lavish love. In Your most holy name I pray. Amen.

don't keep it to yourself

Congratulations on finishing this workbook! You are well on your way to winning the battle for sexual and emotional integrity. I pray that you have learned how to guard not just your body, but also your mind, heart, and mouth from sexual compromise. I pray you have discovered God's plan for ultimate sexual fulfillment. But most of all, I hope you have tasted and seen that, in fact, the Lord is good and His plans are perfect.

If you've just completed *Every Single Woman's Battle* on your own and benefited from it, let me encourage you to consider getting a group of other women together and leading them toward discovering God's plan for sexual and emotional fulfillment as well. This can help keep you accountable, but it will also enable you to encourage and help other women who are in the battle with you. If as women we can encourage one another to open up about our struggles in this area, we will be better able to get the support and help we need.

You'll find more information about starting such a group on pages 1-2 of Questions You May Have About This Workbook.

about the author

Shannon Ethridge is a wife, mother, writer, speaker, lay counselor, and advocate for sexual wholeness. Speaking to youth, college students, and adult women since 1989, she is passionate about instilling sexual values in children at an early age, challenging young people to embrace a life of sexual purity, ministering to women who have looked for love in the wrong places, and challenging all women to make Jesus Christ the primary Love of their life.

Shannon Ethridge Ministries seeks to help those who are struggling with sex, love, and relationship issues, and to equip women with resources to lead growth groups throughout the country and abroad.

A weekly instructor on the Teen Mania Ministries campus, Shannon has been featured numerous times on radio and television programs. She and her husband, Greg, have been married for fifteen years and live in a log cabin among the piney woods of East Texas with their two children, Erin (thirteen) and Matthew (ten).

Shannon Ethridge
Ministries

For speaking engagements or other resources available through Shannon Ethridge Ministries, call 1-800-NEW-LIFE, go to www.shannonethridge.com, or e-mail Shannon at sethridge@shannonethridge.com.

Helping women win the **battle** by **building** a strong **foundation** of **integrity**

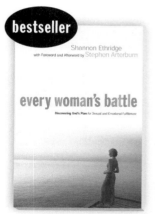

bestseller

Shannon Ethridge
with Foreword and Afterword by Stephen Arterburn

every woman's battle

Discovering God's Plan for Sexual and Emotional Fulfillment

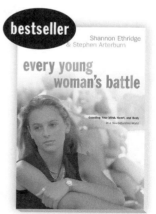

bestseller

Shannon Ethridge
& Stephen Arterburn

every young
woman's battle

Guarding Your Mind, Heart, and Body
in a Sex-Saturated World

Companion workbooks are also available.

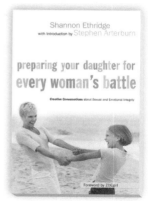

Shannon Ethridge
with Introduction by Stephen Arterburn

preparing your daughter for
every woman's battle

Creative Conversations about Sexual and Emotional Integrity

Foreword by ZOEgirl

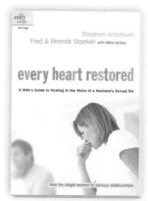

Stephen Arterburn
Fred & Brenda Stoeker with Mike Yorkey

every heart restored

A Wife's Guide to Healing in the Wake of a Husband's Sexual Sin

Also for single women in serious relationships

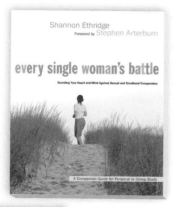

Shannon Ethridge
Foreword by Stephen Arterburn

every single woman's battle

Guarding Your Heart and Mind Against Sexual and Emotional Compromise

A Companion Guide for Personal or Group Study

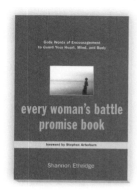

God's Words of Encouragement
to Guard Your Heart, Mind, and Body

every woman's battle
promise book

foreword by Stephen Arterburn

Shannon Ethridge

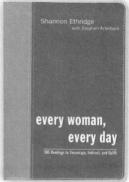

Shannon Ethridge
with Stephen Arterburn

every woman,
every day

365 Readings to Encourage, Instruct, and Uplift

Available in bookstores everywhere.

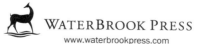
WATERBROOK PRESS
www.waterbrookpress.com

Now Available from Shannon Ethridge Ministries

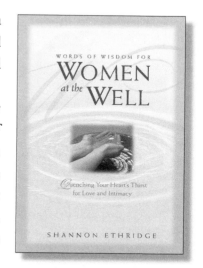

Does your thirst for love and intimacy seem insatiable? Are you choking on the bitter taste of broken relationships or sexual struggles? Are you ready to taste the Living Water that Jesus offered the Woman at the Well so that she would "never thirst again?"

Experiencing the lavish love of God for yourself is the only way to quench your deep thirst for love and intimacy. *Words of Wisdom for Women at the Well* can help you: recognize the "neon sign" that draws unhealthy men your direction, identify the core issues that pull you into dysfunctional relationships, surrender guilt and shame that lead you to medicate your pain with men, discover the "heavenly affair" that the Lord passionately draws us into, and prepare for stronger, healthier relationships in the future.

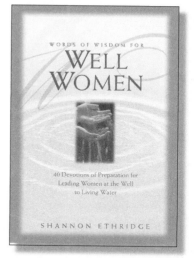

Once you've tasted the Living Water that Jesus offers, you'll no longer be a *Woman at the Well*, but a *Well Woman*!

And more than likely, you'll want to do just as the original Woman at the Well did in Samaria after her intimate encounter with Jesus—invite others to taste the life-changing love of Christ!

Through these forty devotions of preparation, *Words of Wisdom for Well Women* will help you: remain faithful in nurturing your own intimate relationship with Christ, plan and conduct powerful *Well Women* growth group meetings, empower others to live sexually pure and emotionally fulfilling lives, and begin a new kind of sexual revolution in your corner of the world!

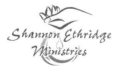

For information on how to order these books
go to www.everywomansbattle.com
or call 1-800-NEW LIFE

the best-selling every man series—for men in hot pursuit of God's best in every area of life

Go beyond easy answers and glib treatments to discover powerful, practical guidance that makes a difference in men's lives—and in their relationships with God, the women in their lives, their friends, and the world.

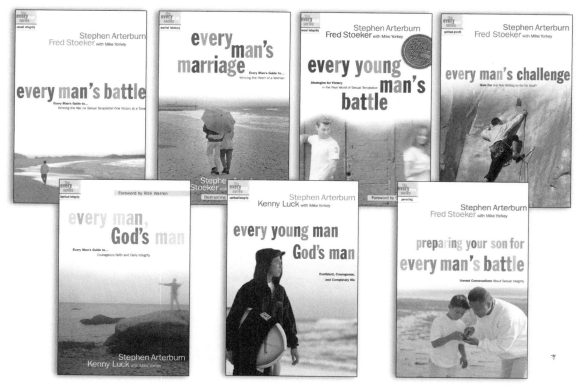

Every Man's Battle
Every Man's Battle Workbook
Every Man's Battle Audio
Every Man's Battle Guide

Every Man's Marriage
Every Man's Marriage Workbook
Every Man's Marriage Audio

Every Young Man's Battle
Every Young Man's Battle Workbook
Every Young Man's Battle Guide
Every Young Man's Battle DVD
Every Young Man's Battle Video

Every Man's Challenge

Every Man, God's Man
Every Man, God's Man Workbook
Every Man, God's Man Audio

Every Young Man, God's Man
Every Young Man, God's Man
 Workbook

Preparing Your Son for Every
Man's Battle

For more information visit www.waterbrookpress.com. Available in bookstores everywhere.

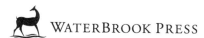

WATERBROOK PRESS